HOLISTIC APPROACHES TO MANAGING AUTOIMMUNE EYE CONDITIONS

Expert Guide to Natural Therapies, Lifestyle Changes, and Wellness Strategies for Optimal Vision Health

DR. CHRIS FRIEDRICH

Disclaimer

This book on Herbal Remedies is intended solely for informational and educational purposes.

The content provided within this book is based on general knowledge and should not be considered as professional advice. The author is not a licensed medical professional, and the information presented here is not intended to diagnose, treat, cure, or prevent any disease.

Readers are advised to consult with qualified healthcare professionals before initiating any herbal remedies or making changes to their existing health regimen. The author and publisher disclaim any responsibility for any adverse effects or consequences resulting from the use of information contained in this book.

It's important to note that the content of this book is not endorsed by any specific platform or affiliated with any product or service.

The author does not receive any compensation or benefits from the promotion of specific herbal products or brands.

Readers should exercise their discretion and judgment when applying the information from this book, and they are encouraged to conduct further research and seek guidance from healthcare professionals to make informed decisions about their health and well-being.

"Holistic Approaches to Managing Autoimmune Eye Conditions" is a thorough manual that covers the complex interactions that occur between holistic health practices and autoimmune eye conditions. The first section of the book gives a comprehensive overview of autoimmune eye conditions, which paves the way for the discussion of holistic approaches that follow. Chapter 1 explores the complexities of several different autoimmune eye conditions, including uveitis, Sjögren's syndrome, ocular myasthenia gravis, and others, elucidating their nuances and emphasizing the necessity of a holistic paradigm.

Chapter 2 provides an overview of the concepts of holistic health and provides a sophisticated analysis of integrative medicine as it relates to autoimmune eye conditions. Chapter 3 delves into the role that diet, vitamins, minerals, and antioxidants play in promoting eye health from an anti-inflammatory perspective, while Chapter 4 explores complementary therapies, mind-body practices, and nutritional approaches.

These chapters highlight the complexity of holistic healthcare.

In Chapter 4, the complex relationship between stress and autoimmune eye conditions is discussed. Mind-body techniques such as yoga, meditation, and breathing exercises are recommended as integral parts of holistic treatment. Chapter 5 delves into herbal and natural remedies, highlighting traditional methods like aloe vera, bilberry extract, and turmeric while combining these with conventional treatments.

This book, with its thorough investigation and useful insights, is an invaluable resource for healthcare professionals, researchers, and anyone looking for a holistic approach to autoimmune eye conditions. Chapter 6 advocates lifestyle changes as essential components of holistic eye health, including the role of exercise, sleep, and environmental factors.

Chapter 7 emphasizes the importance of collaborative care, outlining the process of building a holistic healthcare team and facilitating effective communication with ophthalmologists and specialists. The final Chapter 8 presents real-life case studies and success stories, offering tangible evidence of people managing autoimmune eye conditions successfully through holistic approaches.

First Of All

Since the immune system mistakenly attacks its ocular tissues, autoimmune eye conditions present special challenges for treatment and care. As a result, a comprehensive and holistic approach is required to address not only the symptoms but also the underlying causes and contributing factors.

In this context, the concept of a holistic approach emerges as a promising avenue for effectively managing autoimmune eye conditions. Over time, the management of autoimmune eye conditions has changed significantly due to the growing recognition of the intricate relationship between the immune system and ocular health.

Synopsis Of Autoimmune Ocular Disorders

Autoimmune eye conditions comprise a wide range of disorders, such as scleritis, autoimmune retinopathies, and uveitis. These conditions arise from an abnormal immune response that targets different parts of the eye, causing inflammation, tissue damage, and possibly vision impairment. The development of targeted therapeutic strategies is necessary to address the underlying mechanisms of these conditions. For example, uveitis, which is defined as inflammation of the uvea, calls for a customized approach that takes into account the role of the vascular network and the delicate structures of the eye. Similarly, autoimmune retinopathies occur when the immune system misidentifies retinal proteins, requiring interventions that not only suppress inflammation but also

The Value Of Holistic Methods

The use of holistic approaches in the management of autoimmune eye conditions is becoming more popular because they can address the multifaceted nature of these disorders. Unlike traditional treatments, which may concentrate only on suppressing inflammation, holistic approaches acknowledge the interdependence of various factors influencing ocular health.

These factors include lifestyle, environmental factors, the patient's overall well-being, and the intricate balance of the immune system.

By taking a holistic approach, medical professionals seek to improve patient's overall quality of life and lower their risk of recurrence of the disease. Additionally, holistic approaches recognize the psychosocial impact of autoimmune eye conditions, stressing the significance of

Immunoregulation And Strategies To Reduce Inflammation

Immunomodulation and anti-inflammatory strategies are fundamental to holistic approaches to managing autoimmune eye conditions. While corticosteroids and immunosuppressive agents are often used in traditional treatments to suppress the immune system and reduce inflammation, the holistic approach emphasizes the need for targeted interventions that modulate the immune system without compromising its essential functions.

One such targeted intervention could be the use of biologics, which selectively target specific immune system components, allowing for a more precise and nuanced therapeutic approach.

Knowing the immunological subtleties of autoimmune eye conditions helps healthcare providers customize treatment regimens, minimizing side effects and optimizing outcomes.

Dietary Interventions And Lifestyle Adjustments

Holistic management acknowledges the influence of lifestyle and nutrition on immune function and overall health. Antioxidant-rich diets, including vitamins A, C, and E, have been linked to anti-inflammatory effects and may help mitigate autoimmune responses.

Omega-3 fatty acids, which are found in fish oil, have anti-inflammatory properties and may help manage certain autoimmune eye conditions. Lifestyle changes, such as consistent exercise, stress reduction, and getting enough sleep, are essential parts of holistic approaches.

These lifestyle factors not only improve overall health but also influence immune function and may have an impact on immune function.

Patient Empowerment And Education

Understanding the psychosocial aspects of living with autoimmune eye conditions allows healthcare providers to tailor educational efforts to address the emotional and mental well-being of patients. Empowering patients through education fosters a sense of empowerment and active participation in their healthcare. Patients who are well-informed about their condition, treatment options, and the significance of adherence are more likely to make informed decisions, adhere to treatment regimens, and actively engage in lifestyle modifications. Lastly, holistic approaches prioritize patient education and empowerment as essential components of successful management.

Complementary Medicine And Integrative Therapies

A holistic approach includes complementary and integrative medicine as adjunctive measures in the management of autoimmune eye conditions. Complementary medicine includes herbal supplements and traditional medicine from various cultures; some of these compounds have anti-inflammatory and immunomodulatory properties.

Integrative therapies, like acupuncture and chiropractic care, may provide additional benefits in terms of symptom relief and overall well-being; evidence for the efficacy of these therapies in autoimmune eye conditions is evolving, but their role as complementary options in a holistic framework is increasingly recognized.

Considering Psychosocial Support And Mental Health

The psychosocial consequences of autoimmune eye conditions are significant, and holistic approaches place a high value on psychosocial support and mental health considerations.

 Since living with a chronic autoimmune condition that affects vision can cause emotional distress, anxiety, and depression, mental health support should be incorporated into the management plan to address the holistic well-being of individuals with autoimmune eye conditions.

Psychosocial interventions, such as mindfulness-based practices, counseling, and support groups, can enhance resilience and help patients develop coping mechanisms.

A holistic approach to the management of autoimmune eye conditions is a paradigm shift in the understanding and treatment of these complex disorders. Healthcare professionals can create comprehensive strategies that go beyond symptom control by acknowledging the multifaceted nature of these conditions.

The pillars of holistic management include immunomodulation, nutritional interventions, lifestyle modifications, patient education, integrative therapies, and psychosocial support. Adopting this holistic paradigm improves clinical outcomes as well as the general well-being of people with autoimmune eye conditions.

As research continues to uncover the intricate mechanisms of these disorders, the holistic approach offers a dynamic and patient-centered approach to managing autoimmune eye conditions.

CHAPTER ONE
UNDERSTANDING AUTOIMMUNE EYE CONDITIONS

The term "autoimmune eye conditions" refers to a group of diseases in which the immune system mis attacks healthy cells in the eyes, resulting in inflammation and a variety of symptoms. Uveitis, Sjögren's Syndrome, ocular myasthenia gravis, and a few other conditions are common autoimmune eye conditions that can have a substantial impact on visual function and overall ocular health. Uveitis is a common autoimmune condition that is characterized by inflammation of the uvea; Sjögren's Syndrome, on the other hand, primarily affects the moisture-producing glands, causing dry eyes and other systemic manifestations; and ocular myasthenia gravis is a neuromuscular disorder that affects eye movement.

The variety of these conditions calls for a thorough and integrative approach

Reasons And Initiators

The genesis of autoimmune eye disorders is complex and involves genetic, environmental, and immunological factors. Genetic factors are important because some people are born with a predisposition to autoimmune disorders; knowing the genetic basis of these conditions can help with early diagnosis and customized treatment plans. Environmental factors include exposure to certain toxins or infections, which can act as triggers for autoimmune responses in susceptible individuals. Finally, immunological factors have a major role in the development of autoimmune eye disorders because they cause tissue damage and chronic inflammation when the immune system misinterprets ocular tissues as foreign.

Comprehensive Methods For Managing

A holistic approach is essential to the management of autoimmune eye conditions because of the complex nature of these disorders.

To achieve comprehensive and effective care, a holistic approach integrates medical, lifestyle, and psychological considerations. Medical interventions typically involve immunosuppressive medications, corticosteroids, and anti-inflammatory drugs to control the immune response and alleviate symptoms. However, a holistic approach goes beyond pharmacological treatments and incorporates lifestyle modifications to improve overall well-being. These adjustments could involve stress reduction methods, consistent exercise, and dietary adjustments.

All of these things can positively influence the immune system and aid in the overall management of autoimmune eye conditions.

Genetic Elements

An individual's susceptibility to uveitis and other autoimmune disorders is largely determined by their genetic predisposition, and knowledge of the specific genes involved can help identify those who are at a higher risk and implement early interventions. Genetic testing can be used to determine an individual's risk profile and assist healthcare providers in customizing treatment plans.

Furthermore, advances in genetic research may lead to targeted therapies that address the underlying genetic factors contributing to autoimmune eye conditions, which would be a significant step toward personalized medicine in ophthalmology.

Environmental Elements

A holistic management approach necessitates the identification and mitigation of environmental triggers for autoimmune eye conditions. Infections, like bacterial or viral conjunctivitis, can act as catalysts for the immune system's aberrant response, causing inflammation in the eyes; exposure to environmental toxins, like pollutants or certain chemicals, has also been linked to the development of autoimmune disorders; and patient education about protective measures, like proper hygiene and avoiding known environmental triggers, becomes essential in preventing flare-ups and maintaining ocular health.

Immunological Elements

Immunomodulatory therapies, such as immunosuppressive medications and biologics, are commonly used to modulate the immune response and alleviate symptoms of autoimmune eye conditions. However, a holistic approach recognizes the importance of balancing immune suppression with maintaining the body's ability to defend against infections. Monitoring immune function and customizing immunomodulatory treatments to individual responses are critical considerations in managing autoimmune eye conditions from an immunologic perspective.

This dysregulation of the immune system results in chronic inflammation and tissue damage, characteristic of conditions like uveitis and Sjögren's Syndrome.

As research continues to uncover the complexities of these conditions, a holistic approach to managing autoimmune eye conditions is essential for providing comprehensive care that takes into account the variety of factors that contribute to these disorders.

Knowing the specific autoimmune eye conditions, their causes, and how genetic, environmental, and immunological factors interact allows healthcare professionals to create individualized treatment plans that are both effective and personalized.

The cornerstone of holistic management is a combination of medical interventions, lifestyle modifications, and psychological support, with the goal of not only relieving symptoms but also improving overall health and quality of life for those affected by these conditions.

CHAPTER 2
APPLYING HOLISTIC PRINCIPLES TO MANAGE AUTOIMMUNE OCULAR DISORDERS

In the context of treating autoimmune eye disorders, holistic health refers to an all-encompassing strategy that takes into account the interdependence of different facets of a person's health. It goes beyond treating eye symptoms and targets the underlying causes of autoimmune disorders that affect the eyes. Holistic health emphasizes the integration of physical, mental, emotional, and spiritual dimensions to support general harmony and balance within the body.

Autoimmune Eye Disorders And Integrative Medicine

To maximize the efficacy of standard medical interventions while minimizing side effects, integrative medicine plays a critical role in the management of autoimmune eye conditions by combining conventional medical treatments with complementary and alternative approaches.

When it comes to autoimmune eye conditions, integrative medicine emphasizes the significance of taking the individual's unique circumstances into account and customizing treatment plans accordingly.

Alternative Medicine

Acupuncture, herbal medicine, chiropractic adjustments, massage therapy, and other non-traditional therapies are examples of complementary therapies that complement conventional medical interventions in the management of autoimmune eye conditions. These therapies are chosen for their ability to address particular symptoms, reduce medication side effects, and improve the general health of the patient.

Complementary therapies also seek to produce a synergistic effect that strengthens the body's natural healing and homeostasis.

Mind-Body Techniques

The integration of mind-body practices—such as meditation, yoga, and mindfulness—into the holistic management of autoimmune eye conditions is important. Mind-body techniques aim to reduce stress, which is known to trigger autoimmune responses. By fostering emotional well-being and relaxation, mind-body practices create an environment that is more conducive to the body's ability to regulate its immune system, potentially mitigating the severity of autoimmune eye conditions and supporting overall ocular health.

Dietary Methods

To support ocular health, specific dietary components, such as omega-3 fatty acids, antioxidants, and anti-inflammatory foods, may be emphasized. Nutritional strategies also take into account potential food sensitivities or allergies that could exacerbate autoimmune responses. Individuals can work with healthcare professionals to customize their diets to address specific needs and optimize their overall health, potentially influencing the course of autoimmune eye conditions. Nutritional approaches are fundamental to the holistic management of autoimmune eye conditions.

Finally, holistic approaches to the management of autoimmune eye conditions involve a complex approach that incorporates multiple holistic health principles. Integrative medicine, which includes complementary therapies, mind-body practices, and nutritional approaches, acknowledges the significance of treating the patient as a whole, taking into account physical, mental, emotional, and spiritual aspects. This all-encompassing approach seeks to maximize the effectiveness of traditional medical treatments while fostering general well-being and reducing side effects. As our understanding of autoimmune disorders advances, incorporating holistic principles into eye care offers a promising path to better outcomes and a higher quality of life for those who suffer from autoimmune eye conditions.

CHAPTER 3
DIET AND NUTRITION FOR OCULAR HEALTH

Understanding the complex relationship between nutrition and the immune system is crucial to the holistic management of autoimmune eye conditions. Nutrition plays a role in autoimmune conditions that go beyond simple sustenance and involve a complex interplay with the body's immune response. Numerous studies have shown the influence of dietary choices on the modulation of immune functions, indicating that a customized nutritional approach can be a useful adjunct in the management of autoimmune eye conditions. Understanding the importance of nutrition requires examining particular dietary components, such as macronutrients and micronutrients, that are critical to maintaining ocular health.

A Diet Low In Inflammation

A key component of treating autoimmune eye diseases is implementing an anti-inflammatory diet. As autoimmune disorders are characterized by chronic inflammation, dietary interventions can impact the inflammatory response.

Omega-3 fatty acids, which are abundant in fatty fish such as salmon and flaxseeds, have gained recognition for their strong anti-inflammatory qualities. Specifically, eicosapentaenoic acid (EPA) and docosahexaenoic acid (DHA) fatty acids demonstrate immunomodulatory effects that may reduce inflammation related to autoimmune eye diseases.

Fatty Acids Omega-3

When it comes to autoimmune eye conditions, omega-3 fatty acids are particularly important. These fats are not only necessary for good health overall, but they may also be able to help control inflammation. Studies have shown that omega-3 fatty acids can affect immune cell function and cytokine production, which can have an anti-inflammatory effect. Including foods high in omega-3 fatty acids, like flaxseed oil or fish oil supplements, can help maintain a healthy immune system and potentially reduce the symptoms of autoimmune eye conditions.

Minerals And Vitamins

Ensuring an adequate intake of these vitamins and minerals through a well-balanced diet or supplementation may contribute to the holistic management of autoimmune eye conditions by bolstering the body's immune defenses.

Vitamins and minerals are necessary for maintaining the integrity of the ocular surface and overall ocular health. Specific micronutrients, such as vitamins A, C, D, and zinc, have been implicated in modulating immune functions and protecting against inflammation.

Antioxidants

Another essential component of a comprehensive strategy for treating autoimmune eye disorders is antioxidants. Oxidative stress, which is defined as an imbalance between antioxidants and free radicals in the body, has been linked to the pathogenesis of several autoimmune disorders that affect the eyes.

Antioxidants, which are abundant in fruits and vegetables, act as scavengers of free radicals, counteracting their damaging effects. Including a wide variety of foods high in antioxidants, such as nuts, berries, and leafy greens, may protect against oxidative damage and slow down the advancement of autoimmune eye conditions.

Taking a comprehensive approach to the management of autoimmune eye conditions entails having a thorough understanding of the complex interactions that exist between nutrition and the immune system.

Understanding the role that nutrition plays in autoimmune conditions and putting an anti-inflammatory diet that is rich in vitamins, minerals, and antioxidants can improve the general health of people who are dealing with these eye disorders. This subtle nutritional approach, when combined with traditional medical interventions, has the potential to improve the quality of life for people who suffer from autoimmune eye conditions.

CHAPTER 4
STRESS-MANAGEMENT MIND-BODY PRACTICES

The integration of mind-body practices in the treatment of autoimmune eye conditions is emphasized in the holistic approach, which acknowledges the complex relationship between the mind and body and takes into account the influence of psychological factors on the immune system and, in turn, on autoimmune conditions that affect the eyes.

A key idea behind holistic approaches to health is the mind-body connection, which recognizes that mental and emotional states can have a substantial impact on physical health. When it comes to autoimmune eye conditions, stress is recognized as a possible trigger or aggravating factor. Prolonged stress can cause immune system dysregulation, which can increase inflammation and exacerbate symptoms of autoimmune eye diseases.

It is important to comprehend this complex relationship between mental states and physiological responses to develop comprehensive strategies for managing these conditions.

An investigation into the particular stressors that people with autoimmune eye conditions may encounter is necessary to customize interventions that address the underlying causes of stress and foster long-term well-being. Stressors, whether environmental, psychological, or physiological, can trigger the body's stress response, resulting in the release of stress hormones like cortisol.

These hormones, in turn, can modulate immune function, potentially triggering or intensifying autoimmune reactions in the eyes.

The impact of stress on autoimmune eye conditions can be significantly reduced by the use of relaxation techniques. One such technique is meditation, which entails developing mindfulness and awareness through focused attention or guided practices.

Research indicates that consistent meditation practice can have a positive impact on the immune system, lowering inflammation and promoting immune homeostasis overall.

Including mindfulness meditation in the treatment of autoimmune eye conditions may provide people with a useful tool for managing stress and gaining control over their health.

Yoga is another mind-body practice that integrates physical postures, breath control, and meditation to support holistic well-being. Yoga has been investigated as a complementary therapy to improve quality of life and alleviate symptoms in the context of autoimmune eye conditions.

The physical aspect of yoga improves circulation and flexibility, and the meditation component helps reduce stress. Developing a customized yoga practice can offer individuals with autoimmune eye conditions an integrative method of managing their physical and psychological health.

Controlled breathing patterns, such as diaphragmatic breathing or deep belly breathing, have been shown to activate the body's relaxation response, reducing stress and anxiety.

Given the association between stress and autoimmune eye conditions, regular breathing exercises can help reduce stress and potentially modulate the immune response, giving individuals a self-directed tool for improving their overall health. Breathing exercises are a specific subset of relaxation techniques that target the respiratory system to induce a state of calmness and balance.

Ultimately, a comprehensive approach to managing autoimmune eye conditions must acknowledge the complex relationship between the mind and body. Stress, for example, is a major factor that influences the course of autoimmune diseases and must be targeted for mitigation. Mind-body practices, such as yoga, meditation, and breathing exercises, provide individuals with autoimmune eye conditions with useful tools for managing stress and improving their general well-being. When these practices are incorporated into a comprehensive management plan, people can take charge of their health and take action, addressing not only the physical symptoms of their condition but also the underlying psychological factors that are contributing to its progression.

CHAPTER 5
HERBAL AND NATURAL REMEDIES

A wide range of therapeutic strategies are employed in the management of autoimmune eye conditions, and one important component of this paradigm is the investigation of traditional herbal remedies, which acknowledges the potential advantages of medicinal plants in symptom relief and ocular health promotion. Curcumin, the active ingredient in turmeric, has been thoroughly researched for its anti-inflammatory and antioxidant qualities; using turmeric to treat autoimmune eye conditions aims to modulate immune responses and reduce inflammation, offering a natural substitute or adjunct to traditional treatments.

As a traditional herbal remedy, bilberry extract is gaining attention for its potential role in managing autoimmune eye conditions by targeting underlying inflammatory processes.

Rich in anthocyanins and other bioactive compounds, bilberry has demonstrated anti-inflammatory and antioxidant effects, potentially contributing to the protection of ocular tissues. Studies suggest that bilberry may enhance microcirculation and reduce oxidative stress, thereby promoting overall eye health.

While research specific to autoimmune eye conditions is limited, the general anti-inflammatory effects of aloe vera suggest its potential to mitigate ocular inflammation and discomfort. Aloe vera, known for its medicinal properties, is also being explored in the context of holistic management of autoimmune eye conditions. The gel derived from the aloe vera plant contains various bioactive compounds with anti-inflammatory and wound-healing properties. Including aloe vera in holistic treatment plans reflects a holistic perspective that embraces natural remedies as adjuncts to conventional interventions.

A comprehensive strategy that combines the best aspects of both paradigms is the integration of natural remedies with conventional treatments. This approach acknowledges the potential synergies between herbal/natural remedies and established medical interventions, to optimize therapeutic outcomes. For example, the integration of herbal supplements into treatment regimens may improve the overall efficacy of conventional medications.

 The integrative approach also takes into account the complexity of autoimmune eye conditions and addresses various aspects of the disease, such as inflammation, oxidative stress, and immune dysregulation.

the comprehensive management of autoimmune eye conditions entails a nuanced investigation of different herbal and natural remedies. Herbal approaches, like those involving aloe vera, turmeric, and bilberry extract, present promising avenues for promoting ocular health and mitigating inflammation. The combination of these natural remedies with conventional treatments is a progressive tactic that capitalizes on the advantages of both paradigms to provide comprehensive and individualized care for patients with autoimmune eye conditions. This holistic approach emphasizes the significance of taking into account the variety of therapeutic options that are available and customizing treatment plans to each patient's specific requirements.

CHAPTER 6
CHANGES IN LIFESTYLE FOR EYE HEALTH IN

A comprehensive strategy for managing autoimmune eye conditions includes several lifestyle changes that support overall ocular health. One of the most important changes is making exercise and physical activity a regular part of one's routine. Studies have shown that moderate-intensity exercise is associated with better systemic health and that physical activity and reduced inflammation are positively correlated, which is important when it comes to autoimmune conditions that affect the eyes.

Exercise also improves blood circulation, which may slow the advancement of autoimmune-related eye disorders by improving oxygenation and nutrient delivery to ocular tissues.

Implementing practices like keeping a consistent sleep schedule, setting up a conducive sleep environment, and practicing relaxation techniques can support immune system function and contribute to overall ocular health.

Sleep and circadian rhythms play a pivotal role in maintaining immune system balance, and disruptions in these patterns have been linked to an increased susceptibility to autoimmune diseases. Sleep disturbances can exacerbate inflammation, potentially triggering or worsening autoimmune eye conditions. Therefore, adopting healthy sleep habits and addressing circadian rhythm disruptions may be essential components of a holistic management strategy.

Environmental factors have a significant impact on eye health, especially when it comes to autoimmune conditions. Pollution, allergens, and irritants are examples of environmental stressors that can exacerbate inflammation and contribute to the development or progression of autoimmune eye disorders. Taking steps to reduce exposure to these factors, such as wearing protective eyewear, using air purifiers, and creating a space free of allergens, can be crucial to managing autoimmune eye conditions holistically. It is also important to take into account the impact of lifestyle choices like smoking on eye health, as smoking has been linked to increased inflammation and a higher risk of autoimmune diseases that affect the eyes.

a comprehensive strategy for managing autoimmune eye disorders must include lifestyle modifications. Physical activity enhances general health and lowers inflammation, while immune system function is supported by proper sleep patterns and addressing circadian disruptions. Environmental factors, such as reducing stress and forming healthy habits, also have a substantial impact on the general well-being of people with autoimmune-related eye disorders.

Nutritional Therapies For Autoimmune Eye Disorders

A well-tailored diet is essential for managing autoimmune eye conditions, as nutrition plays a major role in both disease progression and symptom severity. Diet and autoimmune disorders, including ocular autoimmune disorders, are complex, and the individual's condition will determine the specific dietary interventions needed; however, general guidelines can help with dietary modifications for a comprehensive approach to managing autoimmune eye conditions.

For people with autoimmune eye disorders, an anti-inflammatory diet can be helpful. Foods high in omega-3 fatty acids, like walnuts, flaxseeds, and fatty fish, have been linked to decreased inflammation and better symptoms of autoimmune diseases. Foods high in antioxidants, like fruits, vegetables, and green tea, can also help to reduce oxidative stress, which is a common aspect of autoimmune eye disorders. Finally, keeping a well-balanced diet that provides a range of nutrients is essential for sustaining immune system function in general.

Some people with autoimmune conditions find relief from symptoms by identifying and avoiding specific foods that may exacerbate inflammation or trigger immune responses. Common triggers include gluten, dairy, and certain nightshade vegetables. It is important to approach elimination diets under the guidance of healthcare providers to ensure nutritional adequacy and prevent unintended consequences. Elimination diets, such as removing potential trigger foods, may be explored in consultation with healthcare professionals.

A comprehensive dietary strategy may also include supplementation. Specific vitamins and minerals, like zinc, and vitamins A, and D, are important for immune system support and ocular health, but individual needs vary, so supplementation should be customized for each person. Working with healthcare providers, such as dietitians and nutritionists, is essential to creating individualized diet plans that meet the special needs of people with autoimmune eye conditions.

 dietary interventions are essential to a comprehensive approach to managing autoimmune eye conditions. Stressing anti-inflammatory foods, cautiously investigating elimination diets, and taking into account targeted supplementation can improve general health and aid the immune system in controlling autoimmune reactions that impact the eyes.

Psychosocial Support And Stress Reduction In Autoimmune Eye Disorders

Because of the complex relationship between stress and autoimmune eye conditions, a comprehensive approach involving both stress management and psychosocial support is necessary. Chronic stress has been linked to immune system dysregulation and inflammation, which can exacerbate autoimmune diseases, including ocular autoimmune diseases.

For this reason, integrating effective stress management techniques into the overall care plan is crucial for patients with autoimmune-related eye disorders.

In addition, mindfulness-based stress reduction (MBSR) programs have been linked to improvements in overall well-being and may be helpful for people navigating the challenges of autoimmune diseases affecting the eyes.

Mind-body interventions, like meditation and yoga, have shown promise in reducing stress and promoting relaxation. These practices can positively impact immune function, potentially mitigating the autoimmune response involved in eye conditions.

Recognizing the emotional and psychological toll that having a chronic condition takes, psychosocial support is an essential part of holistic management. Support groups, whether they be in-person or virtual, offer a forum for people to exchange stories, coping mechanisms, and emotional support.

 The camaraderie these groups foster can help people feel better mentally and be more resilient to the difficulties that come with autoimmune eye conditions.

By addressing the psychological aspects of living with a chronic illness, professional counseling, and therapy can further enhance holistic care. Living with uncertainties, lifestyle modifications, and potential visual impairments associated with autoimmune eye conditions can be emotionally taxing, and therapeutic interventions offer a helpful space for people to process and work through these challenges.

A holistic approach to managing autoimmune eye conditions must include stress management and psychosocial support. Mind-body interventions, joining support groups, and getting professional counseling are all part of a comprehensive care plan that takes into account the emotional and physical aspects of living with autoimmune-related eye disorders.

CHAPTER 7
WORKING IN COLLABORATION WITH MEDICAL PROFESSIONALS

The concept of building a holistic healthcare team is foundational to an approach that emphasizes the importance of collaborative care involving a diverse team of healthcare professionals.

An understanding that a team of specialists, including rheumatologists, ophthalmologists, immunologists, and other relevant healthcare professionals, can collectively address the diverse facets of autoimmune eye conditions, emphasizes the importance of collaborative care involving a multidisciplinary team of healthcare professionals. This multidisciplinary approach recognizes that autoimmune eye conditions often involve complex interactions between various bodily systems, necessitating expertise from different medical domains.

Putting together a strategic team of professionals with complementary knowledge and skills is the first step in creating a holistic healthcare team. Rheumatologists are essential in treating the underlying autoimmune processes, and ophthalmologists are experts in the complexities of eye health. Immunologists give valuable insights into the immunological aspects of the condition by understanding and modulating the immune system. Allied healthcare professionals, such as nurses and physiotherapists, can also contribute to holistic patient care by treating conditions like rehabilitation, patient education, and general well-being. The synergy created by a cohesive healthcare team guarantees that patients receive thorough and well-coordinated care that goes beyond treatment for their condition.

Another crucial component of the holistic approach is communication with ophthalmologists and specialists.

Good communication within the healthcare team is necessary for information exchange, strategy discussions, and a cohesive approach to patient care. As leaders in the management of eye conditions, ophthalmologists must effortlessly communicate with rheumatologists and other specialists to comprehend the larger context of the autoimmune processes affecting the eyes.

 Tools that help promote effective communication among team members include shared electronic health records, regular case conferences, and multidisciplinary meetings.

One of the most important steps toward improving the effectiveness of care for autoimmune eye conditions is the integration of holistic approaches into medical treatment plans.

Traditional medical treatments, like immunosuppressive medications, may be essential to managing the underlying autoimmune processes, but a holistic approach acknowledges the importance of complementary therapies and lifestyle modifications. Integrating holistic approaches entails incorporating evidence-based practices, like exercise regimens, stress management strategies, and dietary modifications, into the overall treatment plan.

This comprehensive approach takes into account the patient's overall well-being, acknowledging the interplay between physical and mental health and autoimmune conditions.

In addition, integrating holistic approaches into medical treatment plans empowers and educates patients, who are active participants in their healthcare journeys and can make informed decisions by understanding how lifestyle factors play a role in managing autoimmune eye conditions. Holistic interventions, like nutritional counseling and mindfulness practices, can be easily incorporated into treatment plans, empowering patients and improving their sense of control over their care.

This integrative approach is in line with the principles of patient-centered care, which acknowledges the individuality of each patient and customizes treatment plans to meet their specific requirements and preferences.

the implementation of a holistic approach to the management of autoimmune eye conditions is predicated on the cooperative efforts of a heterogeneous healthcare team.

Establishing a Holistic Healthcare Team unites experts from multiple disciplines, each of whom contributes their knowledge to tackle the intricacy of autoimmune processes impacting the eyes. Skillful Communication with Ophthalmologists and Specialists guarantees smooth information flow, promoting a cohesive approach to patient care. Including Holistic Approaches in Medical Treatment Plans acknowledges the importance of complementary therapies and lifestyle modifications, thereby boosting the overall effectiveness of treatment. This all-inclusive care model not only addresses the symptoms of autoimmune eye conditions but also considers the patient's overall health.

CHAPTER EIGHT
CASE STUDIES AND SUCCESS STORIES

When it comes to the field of holistic management of autoimmune eye conditions, case studies and success stories are essential for providing light on the effectiveness of these approaches.

These accounts offer priceless insights into the lives of people who have decided to manage their autoimmune eye conditions holistically.

By examining the particulars of these cases, researchers and medical professionals can gain a more comprehensive understanding of the wide range of autoimmune eye conditions, their symptoms, and the various strategies that patients have used.

Analyzing real-world case studies of people who have managed autoimmune eye conditions holistically reveals a range of strategies that go beyond conventional medical interventions.

These case studies frequently highlight the complex interactions between dietary adjustments, lifestyle modifications, and complementary therapies in reducing the symptoms of autoimmune eye disorders.

Knowing the background, obstacles, and victories of people who have undertaken this holistic journey can help medical professionals customize treatment plans for their patients.

Comprehensive examinations of individual cases can delve into how variables like stress reduction, dietary modifications, and complementary therapies lead to better results. For example, a case study could demonstrate the benefits of mind-body techniques like yoga or meditation in lowering inflammation and improving general health. Success stories can shed light on the importance of patient participation, self-advocacy, and the integration of complementary therapies into an all-encompassing treatment plan.

Through the documentation and dissemination of these case studies, the medical community can establish a body of evidence supporting the effectiveness of holistic approaches in the management of autoimmune eye conditions. Researchers can also identify patterns and trends among successful cases, which could guide the creation of evidence-based guidelines for holistic interventions. Finally, these stories provide hope and resilience to those who are dealing with autoimmune eye conditions.

CONCLUSION

When concluding holistic approaches to managing autoimmune eye conditions, it is necessary to summarize the most important findings from an examination of real-world experiences and success stories. Holistic approaches, which include dietary adjustments, lifestyle modifications, and complementary therapies, have become important components of the holistic management of autoimmune eye disorders. The data from case studies illustrates how these approaches are complex and how different factors interact to produce different outcomes.

A personalized and integrative healthcare paradigm is required, as highlighted by the holistic approaches. The one-size-fits-all model is inadequate to address the particular challenges presented by autoimmune eye conditions; instead, a customized approach that takes into account the unique manifestations, triggers, and responses of each patient becomes critical.

Holistic strategies, based on real-world experiences, frequently combine conventional medical treatments with alternative interventions, highlighting the significance of a collaborative and patient-centered approach.

Encouraging People With Autoimmune Eye Disorders

The foundation of holistic healthcare is empowerment, and autoimmune eye conditions are no different. Treating these conditions holistically entails not only treating the physical symptoms but also fostering the psychological and emotional health of individuals.

By educating and empowering patients to take an active role in their healthcare, doctors can make better decisions, patients will adhere to their treatment plans more closely, and overall results will be enhanced.

Giving people with autoimmune eye conditions the information and resources they need to make dietary and lifestyle decisions that promote their health is essential. Education campaigns can address the effects of stress, nutrition, and environmental factors on autoimmune conditions. By recognizing the connections between these factors, patients can make decisions that support their comprehensive treatment regimens.

Additionally, empowerment entails developing a cooperative relationship between patients and healthcare professionals. Promoting candid communication, active engagement in treatment discussions, and shared decision-making fosters individual agency.

This collaborative model acknowledges the distinct experiences and preferences of every patient, recognizing that personalized holistic approaches yield the best results.

The exploration of case studies and success stories reveals the complex tapestry of holistic strategies, highlighting the synergy between complementary interventions and conventional medical treatments.

Ultimately, empowering individuals in their healthcare journeys completes the holistic paradigm, highlighting the significance of education, collaboration, and personalized approaches to foster resilience and well-being in the face of autoimmune eye conditions.

In summary, holistic approaches to managing autoimmune eye conditions are not only viable but also hold immense potential for enhancing the quality of life for affected individuals.